Dr. med. Andreas Ganz
Bernhard Johannes Schmidt

PLAINTEXT compact

The ASPERGER Syndrome

Not only
for Psychotherapists

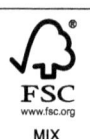

Dr. med. Andreas Ganz
Bernhard J. Schmidt

PLAINTEXT compact
The ASPERGER Syndrome
Not only for Psychotherapists

© 2016 Bernhard J. Schmidt,
Bad Reichenhall, Germany
All Rights reserved.

ISBN: 978 3741276231

translated from
KLARTEXT kompakt
Das ASPERGER Syndrom- nicht nur für Psychotherapeuten
© 2016 Bernhard J. Schmidt
ISBN: 978 383 914 1380
by Klaus Michael Höltershinken

Production and Publishing:
BoD – Books on Demand, Norderstedt, Germany

Bibliographic information of the German National Library:
The German National Library lists this publication
in the German National Bibliography; detailed bibliographic
Data are available online at http://dnb.dnb.de.

Talk with Autistic – not about Autistic!

Research with Autistic – not about Autistic!

Plan with Autistic – not over Autistic!

for
Heidemarie and Albrecht

Table of Contents

I. Preamble 9

II. Introduction 11

III. Autism – Theory 13

   1 Autism - nor treatable, neither a disease!..........14

   2 Sensory Characteristics....................................17

   3 Interpersonal instead of Intrapersonal..............19

   4 Social Psychological Perspective.....................20

      4.1 Unconscious Group Communication / Autopilot_____21
      4.2 Default Mode/Task Mode_____23
      4.3 Without „Autopilot" _____26
      4.4 Without Unconscious Group Communication _____27
      4.5 Summary_____28

   5 Development Dynamic Model..........................29

IV. Genesis of Psycho Structures 32

   1 Seligman „Learned Helplessness"....................32

      1.1 Unpredictability_____34
      1.2 Uncontrollability_____35
      1.3 Helplessness_____35
      1.4 Motivational Consequences_____36

   2 Antonovsky „Salutogenesis"............................37

      2.1 Health Continuum_____37
      2.2 Load Balance_____38
      2.3 SOC – Sense of Coherence _____38

- 2.3.a Comprehensibility...................39
- 2.3.b Manageability........................40
- 2.3.c Significance............................42
- 3 Diathesis-Stress-Model......................................43
  - 3.1 Stage 1: Target _____ 44
    - 3.1.a Possible Stressors...................45
  - 3.2 Stage 0: Complete Retreat _____ 46
  - 3.3 Stage 2: Anxiety and Stress _____ 47
  - 3.4 Consequences: _____ 48
    - 3.4.a „Rejection Sensitivity"...........49
    - 3.4.b Anxiety Disorders...................50
    - 3.4.c Depressive Disorders and Suicide.....51
  - 3.5 Stage 3: Trauma _____ 51
- 4 Consequences...53
  - 4.1 PTSD _____ 54
  - 4.2 Dissociative Personality Structure ____ 57
    - 4.2.a Interaction in Internal Relationships..58
    - 4.2.b Mediated Interaction..............59
    - 4.2.c Interaction in external relationships...60
    - 4.2.d Consequences........................61
  - 4.3 Narcissistic Personality Structure _____ 62

V. Psychotherapeutic Practice 67

- 1 Accessibility..68
  - 1.1 Appointment by Email _____ 69
  - 1.2 Consideration of Hypersensitivity ____ 69
    - 1.2.a Visual......................................70
    - 1.2.b Auditory..................................70
    - 1.2.c Olfactory.................................70
  - 1.3 Home Visits _____ 70

- 2 Anamnesis and Diagnosis..................................71
  - 2.1 With Asperger Diagnosis_____72
  - 2.2 Without Asperger Diagnosis_____73
  - 2.3 SOC Questionnaire_____73
- 3 Psychotherapy Procedures.................................74
- 4 Goals of Therapy..77
  - 4.1 Load Balance – Reduction of Fear and Stress _____77
  - 4.2 Buildup of „Sense of Coherence"_____78
    - 4.2.a Comprehensibility...................79
    - 4.2.b Manageability.........................81
    - 4.2.c Significance............................87
  - 5 Antagonism: „Anxiety Avoiding Behavior".....91
    - 5.1 Avoidance of Change_____92
    - 5.2 Intolerance of Uncertainty_____92
    - 5.3 Insistence on Sameness_____93

VI. Epilogue 94

VII. Appendix 95

  Case Report 1..95

  Case Report 2..100

VIII. Glossary 106

IX. Bibliography 107

I. PREAMBLE

For many decades, the phenomenon autism led a shadowy existence. But in recent years, not only the prevalence sharply increased, but also at least as fast competing or conflicting theories. However, what is missing so far is a "unified theory", a comprehensive explanation as Lynn Waterhouse writes in her book "Rethinking Autism" (Waterhouse 2013).

It needs a theory that can describe not only the causes of (mental) problems, but also the strengths of autistic.

A theory that can explain not only the strong increase in the prevalence of autism, but also the heterogeneity of autistic.

This is particularly necessary for the (psycho-) therapeutic area because many studies in recent years have shown that autistic people have a low HRQL.

In a recent and very large Swedish study (Hirvikoski et al. 2015) now has been shown that autistic people also have a greatly increased risk of mortality.

And as a leading cause of death in people with autism without intellectual impairment suicide is named.

The aim of this book is to provide new approaches for the explanation of the origin of mental disorders in people with autism and hints for the basis for a successful therapeutic treatment.

In this case, the book not only covers the Asperger syndrome, but autism without cognitive impairment in general.

It addresses to psychotherapists and at the same time to people who advising or therapeutically deal in their field of work with autistic.

A corresponding knowledge or training is assumed, which is at least partially necessary for an understanding of the theory presented.

As in the other (German) volumes in this series, the effort to inform compactly prevails.

The interested reader will find the foundations on which this volume incl. its related sources is based in the books "Understanding Autism" (Schmidt 2015/1) and "Assistance for Autistic People?" (Schmidt 2015/2) from the series "Autistic and Society. An angry Change of perspective ".

For recent additions and also and above all a treatment guideline (in German), please see

www.barrierefrei.online

II. INTRODUCTION

The number of different competing theories of Autism is so large that it is impossible to treat them separately in a manageable way. But at least common to the most is that they:

1.) are deficit-oriented,
2.) static in their perception of autism.
3.) Consider autism as an isolated pathological phenomenon.
4.) Do not consider the sensory hypersensitivity.

What distinguishes the approach presented here therefore from traditional approaches? There are mainly five points:

1.) Neuro diversity instead of pathologizing
2.) Consideration of sensory hypersensitivity
3.) Interpersonal instead of Intrapersonal
4.) Social psychology rather than cognition psychology
5.) Development-dynamic model

These new perspectives and the consequences thereof are presented in detail below.

As a result of a development dynamic vision also the need for a diathesis-stress model for the explanation of the emergence of mental disorders in autistic is obvious. Due to the new socio-psychological, also as well as development-dynamic view, a new light falls on previous theories which, inter alia by supplementing to social-psychological insights can serve very well to the understanding of autism. Represented here by way of example with reference to the theory of "learned helplessness" by Martin E. P. Seligman (1975) and the "Salutogenesis" by Aaron Antonovsky (1997).

III. AUTISM – THEORY

Although the individual components of the new Autism theory hereafter are shown separately, they belong together and result from each other. If the beginning is the taking seriously of a "developmental disorder", necessarily actually follows a development-dynamic approach. Together with this even necessarily occurs the consideration of the interaction with the socio-cultural environment.

But that would also result from the diagnostic criteria of autism as an "impairment of INTERaction and COMMUNication".

The foundation for both understanding and therapy of autistic is to leave the current pathologizing and deficit-oriented view. But this view seems to be highly persistent, because as early as 1999 Gray and Attwood wrote in "The discovery of Aspie":

„From Arrogance to Concession and Acceptance
"Without wishing to criticize or point fingers to anyone - typical people are socially arrogant. It seems to be into their very nature, something for which they are not to blame. Proof: Typical people are fascinated by - and concerned about - anyone who is not totally in love with

or excited by their invitations to conversations or games. How can that be?
Typical people see themselves as priceless social occasions; of course everyone should be delighted to be a partner of their interaction. Provided he is normal."

In the professional consideration of autism this until now has unfortunately changed little. And still "cannot" of autistic (due to another way of being) is confused with "does not want" - and this to the detriment of autistic.

1 Autism - nor treatable, neither a disease!

Autism is not a disease but a special form of communication and perception!
So far largely unregarded or even rejected as a myth, is the sensory hypersensitivity of autistic. But especially the hypersensitivity of autistic is, as will be set out, often the cause of e.g. phobias. Here, however hypersensitivity is only about 30% of the cause of the emergence of mental health problems in people with autism.
However, the central diagnostic differentiator is the **impairment of the unconscious group communication!**

With the shift towards "autism spectrum" a big step has been done. But it is unfortunately omitted to think across the pathological border. The deficit-oriented and pathological point of view can overlook healthy autistic. Therefore the autistic with an adequate personal development and without morbidities leading a largely normal life integrated into the community. But precisely these autistic can and should be seen as a target of therapeutic activity. Therefore not a sickening maximum adaptation to the norms of society, but the development of strengths and capabilities, and support, especially in the socio-emotional development.

So a dichotomous opposition between pathological and healthy is to be avoided. Instead, the salutogenetic approach, with its health-disease continuum (see IV.3).

By acceptance of autism as being different instead of being ill the problems are shifted to no or to a wrong diagnosis!

The previously alleged problem with a false positive diagnosis depicts Wilczek:

„It is important to remember that autism is considered "incurable" or "not influenceable by psychotherapy", so that, by a false-positive diagnosis possible intervention may be disregarded, that could effectively reduce or even purposefully resolve symptoms."
[Wilczek 2015]

The perspective of neuro-diversity leads to a distinction in autism as indeed different, but healthy and thus neither treatable let alone requiring therapy firstly and morbidities (anxiety disorders, depression ...) on the other hand as treatable.
This primarily terminates the helplessness!

Example consultancy:
The mere information in advising autistic that these e.g. are treatable anxiety disorders and not autistic, not treatable problems resulted in dramatic improvements without therapeutic intervention!

But:
The differences in sensory perception as well as communication and interaction, even if they are not pathological, lead despite having the same symptoms in different ways to various, not (longer) adaptive psychic structures.
From this follows at least partially the need for a different therapeutic approach and understanding of the pathogenesis of, for example, anxiety disorders, phobias, depression, ... but also dissociative personality structures in autism.

Also the heterogeneity of autistic requires consideration. Therefore, no general specific instructions are possible, but it may be "only" depicted the etiology and general goals of therapy (e.g. manufacture of load balance, structure of SOC, ...).

2 Sensory Characteristics

Autistic perceive their environment usually much more intense, even painful. On the one hand the perception is much more sensitive, e.g. the auditory domain as by a too loud adjusted hearing aid. Secondly, however, disturbing stimuli are not automatically hidden also mainly due to lack of perception-filters. The "party filter" through which the voice of the conversational partner is filtered out of the ambient noise, is missing as well as the ability, e.g. to distinguish the teacher's voice against any existing class noise.
This hypersensitivity can be found both in the auditory, olfactory, visual as well as tactile perception.

Example consultancy:
In physical education a shirt remains. A student with Asperger syndrome assigns the shirt clearly and correctly to the owner solely by smell.

Unfortunately the possibility that this hypersensitivity is a possible cause of phobias, so far hardly has been taken into account. But because of the very strong, painful and overwhelmingly perceived stimulus a unique experience can already cause a "little Albert" effect.

Example consultancy:
A six year old autistic after a single inhalation of the vapors of a sharp vinegar at the table from there on denied eating at the same table.

Many behaviors especially of autistic children can be understood as response to stimuli around perceived as painful!

Example:
A one-time visit in a department store due to an overwhelming painful sensory experience in auditory, visual as well as olfactory area henceforth can result in denial of entry.

According to Seligman (1975) the unpredictability and the repeated experience of uncontrollability of stimuli lead to the "learned helplessness" and hence to anxiety and stress (see IV.2).

Firstly, anxiety and stress can be the causes of stereotyped and repetitive behaviors, which were previously seen as symptoms of autism (see Schmidt 2015/1).

Secondly, however, the permanent experience of anxiety and stress, and thus of helplessness especially leads to impaired motivation, cognition and emotion (Seligman 1975)!

3 Interpersonal instead of Intrapersonal

So far, autism, despite definition as "impairment of INTERaction and COMMUNication" has been considered only isolated, therefore intra personnel.
But interaction and communication always include at least two sides. Both sides can be involved in the "impairment".
Further learning takes place in a socio-cultural environment and e.g. the development of self-esteem needs social interaction.
Also avoiding anxiety by "anxiety avoidance behavior" is an important goal of group behavior (z.B. Menzies Lyth 1960).

So if autistic people have (mental) problems, they are also and above all depending on the socio-cultural environment. Indeed autism is in some environments an increased vulnerability - mainly in affluent societies. But not e.g. in Christian or Buddhist monasteries.
Because there the sensory input is low and communication very limited. Daily routine and activities are highly

structured and ritualized. In addition there are inter alia frequent synchronous activities such as choral singing and also meditation or contemplation, which have positive impact in terms of reducing stress (see e.g. Schmidt 2015/2).

After the perception of the need for interpersonal perspective, the study of the results of social psychology is inevitable.

4 Social Psychological Perspective

Freud introduced the idea of "narcissistic insults of humanity" and named Copernicus, Darwin and psychoanalysis as triggers of these offenses.

However, a further and perhaps more radical insult are the results of social psychology, which could also be the reason why these up to now have not been respected by the Autism Research.

But the results of social psychology since the 1950s by the studies of inter alia Sherif, Asch, Milgram, Zimbardo through to the current book of John Bargh "Social Psychology and the Unconscious: The Automaticity of Higher Mental Processes" are offensive and unambiguous at the same time!

Neuro Typical people (without autism) behave to a large extent just not aware, rational and autonomous, but rather unconsciously, irrational and depending on the group (also see Schmidt 2015/1).

4.1 Unconscious Group Communication / Autopilot

Hitherto known and undisputed is that autistic people have difficulty firstly with small talk and on the other hand with both the perception and decoding as well as the expression of facial expressions and gestures.
However, it was not noted that exactly these, so gossip (called nobly small talk) as well as facial expressions and gestures serve to the unconscious group communication. Thus, while the communication of neuro typical people (NT people) largely consists of gossip as the basis of the unconscious group communication, this falls away in autism.
Thus, communication of NT people consists of a mixture of gossip and factual information interwoven in this. This mixture is also expected from the opposite, since the proportion of the unconscious group communication through gossip and facial expressions and gestures corresponds to a "social grooming".
Autistic against it lack the unconscious relationship proportion of communication, so communication of autistic
    1.   often is greatly reduced compared to NT-people.

2. often by NT-people is perceived as rude because only pure factual information is transmitted.

New perspective

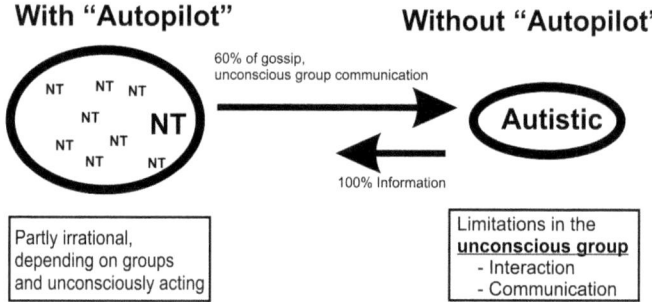

On the other hand autistic find it difficult to filter the relevant content from the "fuzzy" mixture of relationship and factual communications.
This often leads to massive problems in communication. Exclusion, marginalization and harassment of autistic unfortunately often are the consequences (also see Schmidt 2016/2).
Furthermore, unconscious group communication, in which autistic do not participate, also and above all serves as "autopilot", i.e. as an unconscious orientation of the group.

4.2 Default Mode/Task Mode

In the human brain, research by using fMRI (functional magnetic resonance imaging) has identified two different networks, the "Task Positive Network" and the "Default Mode Network". These work like a switch, that is, it can always only one of them be active.

In this case the "Task Positive Network" serves for performing tasks and solving problems.

Contrary the "Default Mode Network" is active if no tasks or challenges are to be tackled.

Derived from this, we distinguish two behavioral states, the

- „Default-Mode" (DM) and the
- „Task-Mode" (TM).

NT people are mostly in DM. This is characterized by:

- unconscious group communication
- gossip, imitation …,
- thus unconscious orientation towards the group,
- resulting superficiality
- and conformity (e.g. in fashion)

The default mode is besides the unconscious communication and interaction especially a power saving mode. Because imitation learning as well as unconscious orientation towards the group consume little energy.

The DM is facing the task-mode (TM). This is, inter alia, marked by:
- Interest instead of superficiality
- Emulation learning rather than imitation(learning)
- Solution orientation instead of group orientation
- High energy consumption (the active brain consumes about 25% of the body's energy, making it as energy consuming as boxing)

Autistic predominantly are in TM! This has several consequences:

1.) AS people lack the "autopilot", i.e. automatic orientation to the group.
2.) They lack the unconscious group communication and interaction, as well as an ingroup / outgroup distinction. Therefore they are often excluded and marginalized, or the target of bullying (see also Schmidt 2016/2).
3.) Due to the lack of "autopilot", the energy requirement is very high.
4.) AS-people do not learn by imitation, but by emulation, i.e. by (repeated) search for own solutions.
5.) AS people communicate only factual information and understand only those.

A juxtaposition of DM and TM as a table:

Default-Mode DM	Task-Mode TM
„Autopilot"	-
power saving mode	energy intensive
imitation learning / overimitation	emulation learning
group-oriented	task and solution oriented
superficiality, gossip	inter-est
▼	▼
NT-People >= 70%	**AS-People** ~ 100%
▼	▼
in-group / out-group	no-group
prejudice	no prejudice
conformity / obedience	heterogeneity
unconscious group-binding	freedom
„pretend play"	-
synchronization	no synchronization

4.3 Without „Autopilot"

The meaning of the autopilot, including the effects of the absence of the unconscious group communication is dependent on the socio-cultural environment!
In a rapidly changing society that is marked by the resolution of clearly defined structures and rituals, the presence of the autopilot as unconscious group orientation is of central importance.

Without autopilot, however, such an environment seems to be not understandable and not predictable - so as uncontrollable both in the sense of Seligman (1975) as well as Antonovsky (1997), to which we shall come back in Chapter IV.

The resulting consequences, which can be seen frequently in people with autism, are:

- „Avoidance of change"
  so avoiding change because changes induce fear.
- „Intolerance of uncertainty"
  so intolerance towards uncertainty.
- „Insistence on sameness"
  and particularly the insistence on equality and resistance.

Three consequences which are also will be considered as resistance to therapeutic intervention.

4.4 Without Unconscious Group Communication

Autistic are unfortunately often, even more and more frequently victims of mobbing and bullying (see also Schmidt 2016/2). And again the socio-psychological point of view provides an explanation of the causes. NT people assign other people automatically either to in-group or out-group (see e.g. Tajfel: minimal group paradigm).

Both the maintenance of group membership as well as the position in the group hierarchy will take place mainly through unconscious group communication! Examples include, inter alia, group-specific clothing styles, dialects (Language does not serve alone the understanding, but also the demarcation!) …

Without unconscious group communication and group orientation thus autistic can neither be assigned to an own group nor a foreign group (!). They are „no-group"! The consequences are:

- Social exclusion
- Marginalization
- Mobbing/Bullying

Group Behavior and Mobbing

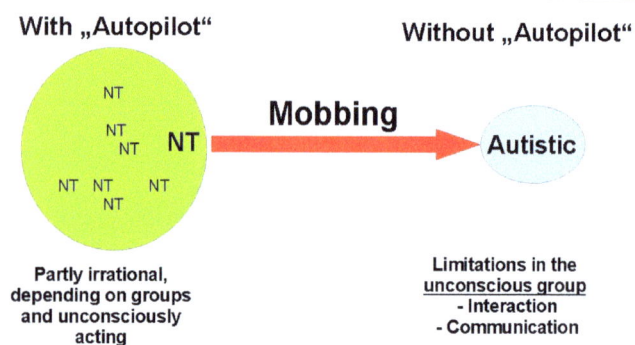

While group membership and group behavior serves NT people also and above all to fear avoidance (see, for example Wetherell, Menzies Lyth), so this also for autistic is not possible because of the lack of unconscious group orientation..

4.5 Summary

As a result of the social-psychological perspective is evident, that

1.) the "impaired social communication and interaction" in fact is a lack of unconscious group communication and interaction!

2.) the cause of the sharp rise in the number of diagnosed autistic is the dramatic change in the socio-cultural environment, i.e. the social environment in regarding

> a) the increase of massive overstimulation.
> b) the elimination of orientation providing structures and rituals.
> c) the permanent change into the DM with corresponding unconscious group orientation.

Autism is therefore not a "pervasive developmental disorder", but may -depending on the socio-cultural environment- result in the disturbance of development, as will be shown in the following.

5   Development Dynamic Model

Despite the previous definition of autism as "pervasive developmental disorder" autism and the resulting problems were regarded statically instead dynamically. But development always is a dynamic process dependent on many factors.

Development Dynamic models have so far been applied to people with mental disabilities, but not to autistic, although autism previously erroneously has been defined as a disability.

"The emergence of special mental health problems of mentally handicapped is developmentally examined, last but not least because in the previous decades, the step from the defect model to development model has taken place. This new way of looking ascribes mentally disabled people the opportunity to develop, with the development steps, phases, and sequences not different from non-disabled."
[Source: de.wikipedia.org „Geistige Behinderung"]

In order to understand autism and to assist autistic therapeutically, it is necessary both to say goodbye to the defect model, as set forth, as well as a development dynamic approach. Without unconscious group orientation, i.e. without autopilot, autistic will develop very differently, so show a large heterogeneity.
In addition, the importance of the socio-cultural environment is made clear by the social-psychological perspective. Thus, a development dynamic perspective is necessary even and especially in autism for understanding the effects of interaction with the environment.

„A development dynamic approach includes mental impairment that can be caused by a malfunction of the social environment." [Source: de.wikipedia.org „Geistige Behinderung"]

Only by means of a dynamic view can ever become obvious how in autism psychological problems arise due to the peculiarities of sensory perception and communication.

IV. GENESIS OF PSYCHO STRUCTURES

The dynamic social psychological perspective sheds new light on existing theories. As examples to this the "learned helplessness" of Seligmann (1975) and the "sense of coherence" of Antonovsky (1997) are presented.

Here, both approaches can and shall not be comprehensively presented but only certain areas by way of example.

Recommended in any case, is the book of Antonovsky (1997), because this also provides a detailed comparison of salutogenesis with other, similar theories.

1   Seligman „Learned Helplessness"

Seligman's approach to learned helplessness is based on the context of the behaviorist stimulus / response paradigm, which may not be surprising because of the time of origin. But against the background of sensory hypersensitivity of autistic, the theory of Seligman is well suited to understand the causes of helplessness, anxiety and stress and depression in people with autism. And the consequent motivational problems.

„...Laboratory experiments on helplessness produce three deficits: they undermine the motivation to respond, they retard the ability to learn that responding works, and they result in emotional disturbance, primarily depression and anxiety." [Seligman 1975]

Why is the concept of "helplessness" helpful in understanding of autism?

„In 1972, D. C. Glass and J. E. Singer reported an extensive series of studies on the role of controllability in reducing stress; they found that merely telling a human subject about controllability duplicates the effects of actual controllability. They attempted to duplicate the stress of the urban environment, by having their subjects —college students—listen to a very loud mélange of sound: two people speaking Spanish, one person speaking Armenian, a mimeograph machine, a calculator, and a typewriter. When subjects could actually turn off the noise by pushing a button, they were more persistent at problem solving, they found the noise less irritating, and they did better at proofreading than yoked subjects." [Seligman 1975]

The stressful situation produced in this experiment by an auditory overload that cannot be turned off, is a continuous experience for autistic due to hypersensitivity

and lack of stimulus filters in a world of overstimulation. And above all, autistic children often lack, unlike the experimental group who could switch off the noise on a button, the ability to terminate a demanding sensory experience.
So the environment is perceived as uncontrollable already in infancy.

„Helplessness in an infant organism has the same consequences as in adults: lack of response initiation, difficulty in seeing that responding works, anxiety, and depression. Since helplessness in an infant, however, is the foundational motivational attitude around which later motivational learning must crystallize, its debilitating consequences will be more catastrophic."
[Seligman 1975]

1.1 Unpredictability

Unpredictability for NT-humans hardly plays a role in the field of sensory perception, because it rarely has a characteristic as overwhelming or painful.
For hypersensitive people, whether autistic or not, this is not true. For them predictability is important as a way of avoiding.

„Unpredictability is the first cousin or uncontrollability; it is defined and related to the previous discussions of helplessness. Predictability is preferred to

unpredictability; stress and anxiety are considerably greater when events occur unpredictably than when they occur predictably, and the behavior of animals and men can be seriously disrupted. More stomach ulcers occur, along with terror and panic." [Seligman 1975]

The unpredictability of (sensory) events so increases anxiety and stress and as a result the likelihood of physiological problems such as stomach ulcers.

1.2 Uncontrollability

If unpleasant or painful (sensory) events cannot be influenced by appropriate behavior, so e.g. loud sounds are turned off, it means that they are uncontrollable.
„When an organism can make no operant response that controls an outcome, I will say the outcome is uncontrollable. " [Seligman 1975]

The combination of unpredictability and uncontrollability then leads to (learned) helplessness.

1.3 Helplessness

The feeling of helplessness arises from the experience of unpredictability and uncontrollability.

„ ...a rigorous definition of the objective circumstances under which helplessness occurs: a person or animal is helpless with respect to some outcome when the outcome occurs independently of all his voluntary responses." [Seligman 1975]

So helplessness is learned and consequently has a large effect on the further behavior.

1.4 Motivational Consequences

The consequences of experienced uncontrollability are massive.
Efforts to respond to further traumatic events at all, e.g. through escape, disappear. However, even if the attempt e.g. of prevention is made and succeeds, it is harder to learn that appropriate responses can be successful.
„Laboratory evidence shows that when an organism has experienced trauma it cannot control, its motivation to respond in the face of later trauma wanes. Moreover, even if it does respond, and the response succeeds in producing relief, it has trouble learning, perceiving, and believing that the response worked. Finally, its emotional balance is disturbed: depression and anxiety, measured in various ways, predominate. The motivational deficits produced by helplessness are in many ways the most striking ..." [Seligman 1975]

Ultimately, depression and anxiety (disorders) may be the consequences as part of a disorder of emotional balance. Thus, using the concept of "learned helplessness" of Seligman shows how for people with autism because of sensory hypersensitivity experiencing and learning of helplessness in a stimulus flooded affluent society is likely.
And how then depression and anxiety disorders can arise as results.

For problems arising from the absence of unconscious group communication, however, the concept of "Salutogenesis" by Antonovsky is better.

2 Antonovsky „Salutogenesis"

The concept of salutogenesis by Antonovsky has three main components. The definition of health as a continuum, the load balance and, especially important for understanding the origin of mental disorders in people with autism, the sense of coherence.

2.1 Health Continuum

For Antonovsky there is no homeostasis, which could be achieved, but only a heterostasis because life always is a process that runs counter to the entropy. Therefore, he also rejects a separation in a "healthy", homeostatic, and a "sick", heterostatic state. For Antonovsky there is a health continuum, on which healthy and sick portions always exist. So the question is only one of the ratio between healthy and diseased portions.

2.2 Load Balance

Life as a rebellion against entropy includes necessary and inevitable the ongoing confrontation with stressors. And these are not only negative, but also necessary for growth and maturation processes. Stressors are therefore not principally the problem, but become such only when they exceed the load limit. This load limit is dynamic and is influenced mainly by the (generalized resistance) resources available.

2.3 SOC – Sense of Coherence

For the development of the theory of the sense of coherence as a factor influencing the development of disease, the finding was crucial that people in a same hostile environment not all are sick. The resulting question what are the causes of the differences in development of the disease as a result of stress, Antonovsky answered with the SOC, the "Sense of coherence".

"I can now redefine the SOC as follows: The SOC (Sense of Coherence) is a global orientation that expresses the extent to which one has a pervasive, persistent and yet dynamic sense of confidence that
1. the stimuli that arise in the course of life from the internal and external environment are structured, predictable and explainable;
2. the resources are available to meet the demands placed by these stimuli;
3. those requirements are challenges that effort and persistence pay off." [Antonovsky 1997]

The three pillars of the SOC are so comprehensibility, manageability and meaningfulness.
In connection with autism therefrom derives the question of whether and to what extent the lack of unconscious group communication and orientation has an influence on the development of comprehensibility, manageability and meaningfulness.

2.3.a Comprehensibility

„Comprehensibility is indeed the well-defined, explicit core of the original definition. It refers to the extent to which one perceives internal and external stimuli as cognitively meaningful, as an ordered, consistent, structured and clear information and not as noise -

chaotic, disorderly, arbitrary, random and inexplicable." [Antonovsky 1997]

It should be noted that Antonovsky did not develop the salutogenesis for a psychotherapeutic context. But already here, at the comprehensibility, with the help of social-psychological perspective becomes obvious, how well the genesis of mental health problems in people with autism can be explained with this concept.
Outside the unconscious group orientation, i.e. without autopilot, the environment seems to be not understandable, to be irrational and arbitrary. And it also largely is, incidentally. It is described by many autistic as "wrong planet" feeling, with the lack of intelligibility can be put into words.

2.3.b Manageability

„ ...this second component manageability and defined it formally as the extent to which one perceives that one has adequate resources available to meet the requirements, emanating from the stimuli to which one is confronted. "Available" are resources that are under self-control, or those that are controlled by legitimate others - spouse, friends, colleagues, God, history, the party leader or a doctor - by someone on whom you can count , someone you trust." [Antonovsky 1997]

Manageability at autism has three sides. On the one hand side of resources mentioned by Antonovsky in the form of friends and colleagues unfortunately often lacking to people with autism. On the contrary, as already shown, autistic (see Schmidt 2016/2) experience more exclusion and bullying than support. Often not only lack the necessary resources to develop the feeling of manageability - it is rather destroyed by the experience of rejection and marginalization.

Another side is that comprehensibility is an important prerequisite for the feeling of manageability:
„It seems clear that a high degree of manageability is highly dependent on a high degree of comprehensibility. A prerequisite for the feeling that one has resources in order to survive against requirements is that one has a clear idea of precisely these requirements. To live in a world that one believes to be chaotic and unpredictable, makes it extremely hard to believe that one gets along well." [Antonovsky 1997]

But as described, it is already missing at comprehensibility as a prerequisite for manageability due to the lack of unconscious group communication. At least in an affluent society in default mode.

The third aspect is the frequent lack of energy due to the missing autopilot.

While NT people with autopilot are comparable to a classic vehicle fully fueled and with reserve indicator as well as replacement canisters autistic rather match an electric car with unreliable charging indicator - and on the highway.

The mere fear that energy suddenly ends and therefore the situation is no longer manageable makes autism sufferers avoid situations that are particularly stressful, so sapping energy and not offering any possibility to retreat.

Example Consultation:
The autistic friend often leaves celebrations suddenly (battery empty) and without saying goodbye. This is perceived by the hosts as unfriendly and rejection.
Further invitations do not happen then.

Although in this example manageability is given by retreat - but still with negative consequences.

2.3.c Significance

,, The third component meaningfulness was also hinted in the original discussion as I warned before of "a strong emphasis on the cognitive aspect of the sense of coherence" (1979, p 127) and pointed how important it is

'to be involved in the processes that make up the own destiny and everyday experience as participant' (S. 128). .... Those who had a strong SOC according to our classification always spoke of areas of life that were important to them which were close to their heart, which 'made sense' in their eyes and that in the emotional not only the cognitive meaning of the term. Events that took place in these areas tended to be viewed as a challenge and as important enough to invest in them emotionally and to get involved." [Antonovsky 1997]

Theoretically, it is of course possible even without the sense of comprehensibility and manageability at least to develop a sense of meaningfulness. But more likely is then the development of a rigid SOC or pseudo-SOC to which we shall return later.

3 Diathesis-Stress-Model

Like the development dynamic perspective although developed for people with intellectual disabilities but not used in autism so it is the same with a diathesis-stress model.
For depression and schizophrenia ... such models do exist – but so far not for autism.
The model developed by us contains four stages, which represent the various forms of stress and trauma and the

resulting problems. This model is, of course greatly simplified, as with all schematic drawings.
Reciprocal effects are many and powerful. That should not be ignored.

3.1 Stage 1: Target

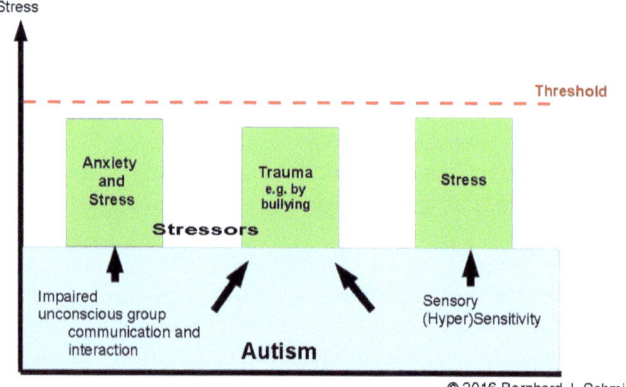

Stage one defines the target whether with or without therapeutic intervention: the load balance. That is, anxiety, stress and trauma in a healthy (!) level exist as a necessary condition of a healthy personality development.

„ … , that a high degree of stress factors with simultaneous high degree of social support is healthy; …" [Antonovsky 1997]

In order to achieve this, either the stressors can be reduced or the threshold increased.

As already stated there are both the sensory hypersensitivity, as well as the deterioration of the unconscious group communication that depending on and interacting with the socio-cultural environment can be a source of anxiety and stress.

Autistic, who are in the load balance, for example, because of good social contacts, a strong sense of comprehensibility, manageability and meaningfulness, i.e. with a high SOC have been ignored simply because they lack the "suffering" necessary for a diagnosis.

3.1.a   Possible Stressors

In addition to stressors also existing at NT-people come in autistic those which arise or are amplified as a result of sensory hypersensitivity, and the absence of unconscious group communication.

1.) „Background Noise"
    a) chronic stressors
    - social conflicts
    - adverse working conditions
    - lack of tasks
    - lack of social contacts

b) everyday stressors
- sensory stress e.g. in (public) traffic
- missing unconscious (group)-orientation, e.g. in purchasing

2.) further stressors
   c) life events
   - disease, bereavement …

   d) systemic stressors
   - fast social change
   - urban anonymity

   e) and for the sake of completeness:
   - catastrophes, floods, earth quake …

3.2 Stage 0: Complete Retreat

Autistic, who have withdrawn completely from the life due to a low SOC and diverse negative experiences, were and are also often overlooked. These barely leave their room (in the family home) or their own home. Although thus stressors and consequently anxiety and stress can be avoided - the health problems such as anxiety disorders and depression not only do not disappear - but become even more massive in most cases..
So retreat is no solution!

Genesis of Psycho Structures

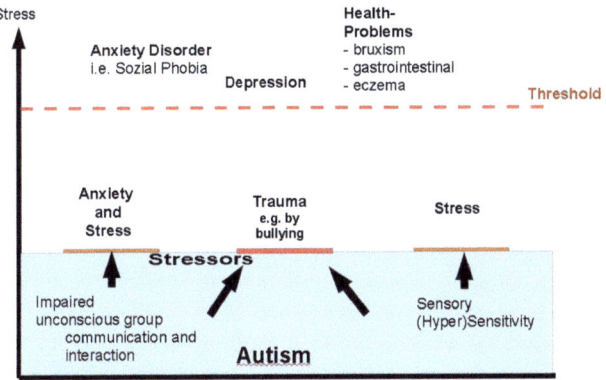

© 2016 Bernhard J. Schmidt

Participation in social (!) interaction and communication is central to mental health and to the development of a healthy personality.

3.3 Stage 2: Anxiety and Stress

At Level 2, the load balance is lost. Stressors produce so much anxiety and stress that the threshold is exceeded. Psychological (anxiety disorders, depression ...) as well as physical (bruxism, gastrointestinal problems, eczema ...) problems are the result. Regarding the development of depressions should be noted that negative automatic thoughts (NAT) in people with autism are also found, but often also permanent real negative experiences by interacting with the environment, by exclusion and marginalization, bullying … Without lowering the real negative experience to a manageable level and simultaneous lifting of the threshold by developing resources therapeutic efforts will remain ineffective.

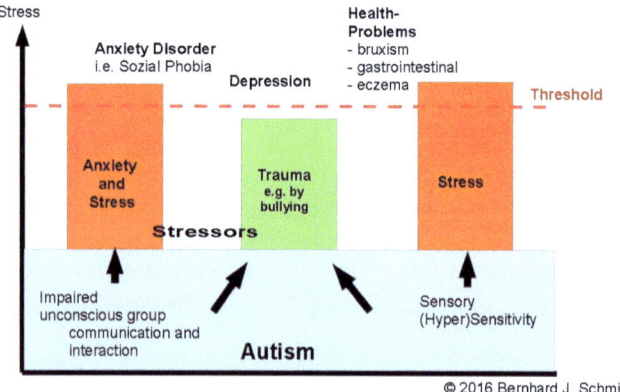

And as has been shown, among other things anxiety and stress are caused by the lack of predictability of the (irrational) group behavior.

3.4 Consequences:

In the field of psychological consequences three are to be discussed in more detail. Rejection sensitivity, anxiety disorder and depressions. Again, there is not the claim of a comprehensive treatment of all aspects. It is, rather, trendsetting ideas for the purposes of road signs.

3.4.a „Rejection Sensitivity"

A central and hitherto ignored point for understanding of autistic and their behavior is the rejection sensitivity. This is hardly available in the scientific perception in German-speaking countries.

Rejection-sensitive are people who anxiously expect rejection, perceive quickly and over-react [Downey (1996)].

This arises from the experience of frequent rejections, which unfortunately are at AS-people's everyday agenda. One factor is the actual rejection by groups due to lack of communication and interaction of unconscious group.

But also due to incorrect, delayed or missing feedback from fellow humans.

Add to that the (false) perception of the irrational (group) behavior of the environment as a rejection.

If one would expect a rational and thus often unambiguous reaction of the opposite, but instead receives a very different one, this can be easily understood as a refusal or rejection.

As a result of experiencing repeated real or imagined rejections then responses and remarks are already perceived as rejection, which were not intended as such.

To these reactions or comments perceived as rejection then will be overreacted due to rejection sensitivity. Either by withdrawal or aggression.

3.4.b   Anxiety Disorders

Anxiety disorders are to be distinguished from (understandable) avoidance behavior. So must e.g. a social phobia be distinguished from avoiding DM-situations. Without unconscious group communication in combination with the lack of small talk, default-mode situations are unpleasant for autistic and either are avoided or transformed into a TM situation.

Example Consultation:
An Asperger student, who otherwise hardly leaves the house, without problems goes from his rural place to an AIDS initiative in the next big city for information about AIDS that he needs for a presentation.

The reshaping of a default mode situation into a task-mode situation therefore is an effective means of participation of autistic in social (!) communication and interaction.

3.4.c Depressive Disorders and Suicide

Depressive disorders require special consideration and attention by all people who professionally work with autistic without intellectual disability!

„People with ASD but without intellectual impairment showed a higher mortality risk by a specific cause: suicide.

'There is a very clear link between ASD without intellectual disability and an increased risk of suicide," said Dr. Hirvikoski. ***'The clinical guidelines for suicidal patients must in any case be followed in individuals with ASD.'***

The study collected data from 27,000 people with ASD, of which 6,400 had an intellectual disability, and about 2.5 million people (adjusted) from the general population."

[PSYLEX.de - Source: Karolinska Institutet, British Journal of Psychiatry; Nov. 2015]

3.5 Stage 3: Trauma

All people suffer traumata. But in people with autism on the one hand, is the probability of traumatic experiences particularly high, on the other hand they often lack the necessary resources for processing. Yes, just those areas that should be the source for the feeling of manageability like friends, colleagues, etc., are either absent or are themselves the source of traumatic experiences, for example, by harassment and bullying - with sometimes dramatic effects on physical and mental health (see also Schmidt 2016/2).

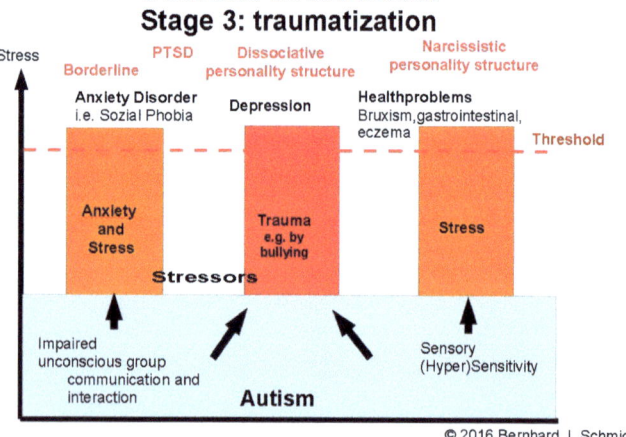

So it is not surprising that there is a not inconsiderable number of autistic have developed corresponding disorders and (formerly adaptive) personality structures like PTSD, borderline personality, dissociative or Narcissistic Personality structure.

Another essential resource, which leads to raising the threshold, is the self-esteem. And this also is based on the communication and interaction with the social environment:

„At the dimension of self-esteem: ... Very important is the self-esteem from the sources of perception and evaluation of one's own performance, powered by the social comparison in cooperation and the consequent evaluation and recognition from the opposite."
[Lorenz 2005]

But this social (!) communication and interaction often is not accomplished with autistic. Instead autistic often experience, as already stated, bullying, exclusion, …
In the Anglo-American countries there are fortunately first changes to the effect that autism no longer is referred to as "disorder, but as "autism spectrum condition (ASC). In Germany, however, autism is still referred to as disorder and autistic thus are additionally stigmatized!

But stigma is detrimental to the development of a healthy self-esteem and in addition also promotes exclusion and marginalization (see also Schmidt 2016/2).

4 Consequences

The possible consequences of stress, anxiety and trauma above the load threshold, are various and cannot all be shown here. So the psychopathological consequences shown in the graph are only a part of possible consequences. Three particularly common and important

consequences nevertheless shall be shortly depicted, again list is not exhaustive:
PTBS, dissociative and narcissistic personality structure.

4.1 PTSD

By the new socio-psychological perspective and the resulting perception of the lack of unconscious communication group two things become obvious:

1. For autistic people, it is difficult to build a high load threshold by interaction with the environment.
2. As "no group" autistic are often ostracized and bullied.

The high risk in people with autism to suffer from PTSD, does not lie, as dell'Osso thinks alone at intrapersonal problems of autistic e.g. a "lack of empathy", but at the exclusion suffered by groups.

„ ...we contemplate current hypotheses that ASD patients are highly susceptible for trauma-related diseases, mainly because of their difficulties in expression, empathy and understanding of common codes of communication that would make them vulnerable to chronic trauma throughout life (King et al., 2010)."
[Dell'Osso et al. 2015]

In addition to a one-time trauma as the cause, not to be treated here, PTSD can also result from repeated traumata. Already at school autistic often are victims of mobbing and bullying. These extend, by definition, over a longer period - and this has dramatic consequences.
„PTSD symptoms can arise from multiple traumata, according to the complex PTSD model (Terr, 1991; Herman, 1992; Van der Kolk, 2005; Hofvander et al, 2009), so to speak, prolonged and / or repeated traumata, such as bullying experiences or repeated sexual abuse. The Complex PTSD symptomatology often is chronic and more severe than typical PTSD symptoms, including deficits in emotion regulation, negative self-perception, interpersonal problems, and dissociative symptoms (King, 2010; Cloitre et al., 2013; Maercker et al., 2013). It was observed that the symptoms of complex PTSD over time lead to long-term instability of interpersonal relationships, emotional lability, unstable self-perception as well as conformist behaviors such as substance abuse and self-injury, so that these clients could be labeled ultimately as borderline patients (King et al., 2010)." [Dell'Osso et al. 2015]

An ongoing trauma of mobbing / bullying can therefore not only result in massive psychological problems - but also lead to a misdiagnosis. Especially with stress and trauma(ta) caused disturbances therefore autism should also be considered and reviewed as underlying vulnerability. As already stated, the overlooking of autism spectrum condition can lead to massive problems in the therapeutic intervention.

„A growing amount of data suggests that individuals with ASD, particularly those with moderate forms without cognitive or linguistic disabilities often only come to clinical attention when other mental disorders occur which lead to challenging diagnostic procedures (Kamio et al, 2013). Sometimes their ASD remains undetected even after the outbreak of these mental illnesses. Takara & Kondo (2014) reported, for example, recently a 16% ASD prevalence among adult depressive patients during the first visit, while Kato et al. (2013) reported rates of 7.3% previously unrecognized ASD in patients hospitalized after attempted suicides. According showed Storch et al. (2013) that suicidal thoughts and actions in adolescents are common with ASD and associated with the presence of depression and PTSD, which seems to suggest that people with ASD represent a group with low resistance and could be especially vulnerable, to develop traumata and stress-related diseases." [Dell'Osso et al. 2015]

Example Clinic:
See Appendix, Case Report 1

In addition to one-time traumatic experiences thus especially the risk of a continuous experience of bullying and exclusion as a possible cause of PTSD is particularly high with autistic. The resulting PTSD symptoms are often chronic and more pronounced. The completion of this enduring traumatic experience e.g. by school bullying has to be accompanied by the therapeutic intervention (see also Schmidt 2016/2).

4.2 Dissociative Personality Structure

A dissociative personality structure, however, is so common and obvious that it is probably for that very reason often overlooked or considered autism typical in people with autism. The published biographies of several autistic very clearly show the separation of normal cognitive and (strongly) reduced social-emotional personality development. But this must not be seen as a necessary and inevitable consequence or accompaniment of autism.

At least two ways can lead to the division of the development of cognition and emotion:
Trauma and a (too) low SOC.

Traumatic experiences as a cause should not be discussed here in order not to carry coals to Newcastle.

Complementing the diathesis-stress model and based on our combination of a dynamic development and socio-psychological approach with the concept of SOC, another way of emergence shall be presented.

The genesis of a DIS on personality development depends on (functioning) communication and interaction with the social environment and has three stages:
1. Interaction in internal relationships
2. Mediated interaction in external relationships
3. Interaction in external relationships

4.2.a Interaction in Internal Relationships

In the first years of life communication and interaction of the child largely happens within the family and with its members. The experience of comprehensibility and manageability is thus directly dependent on the intra-family communication and interaction as well as on family structures.
Firstly, there is the lack of unconscious group communication and of mirroring and synchronization

with the autistic child, which can lead to disorders of the interaction between child and parents.

On the other hand, however, also formerly reliable family structures increasingly dissolve. Starting with the renunciation of family meals to frequently changing life partners, family life is increasingly losing structures and rituals that create or add to the feeling of predictability and manageability in an infant.

4.2.b   Mediated Interaction

If the child is larger, the perception of a mediated communication and interaction with the environment moves into the foreground. So the child's perception of how successful or not the parents or caregivers communicate and interact with the environment. Whether the parents and / or caregivers themselves have a sense of comprehensibility and manageability in contact with the environment, which is conveyed to the child. And if the parents have coping mechanisms that can be learned by the child.

The child assumes, of course, a sense of comprehensibility and manageability already in the internal relationship. If this is not given, then the perception of mediated interaction with the outside world will be difficult.

4.2.c Interaction in external relationships

With the transition into adolescence, it then comes to a gradual detachment from parents, so to leaving the familiar surroundings and the attempt to focus on peers. So the adolescent is trying to get in touch directly with the social environment. And that on the basis of a feeling developed until then of comprehensibility and manageability as well as learned coping mechanisms.

It has already been shown that autistic while lacking both the unconscious group communication as well as the autopilot are facing particular difficulties.

If the SOC or the learned coping mechanisms are insufficient or if the interaction with the social environment is experienced as too traumatic, it does not come to the separation from the family, but to recourse to an ontically upstream behavioral level. The cognitive development then goes on normally, but the socio-emotional development comes to a standstill.

Without leaving the parental home and without establishing positive relations with the social environment, also coping mechanisms independent of the family cannot be learned and the sense of comprehensibility and manageability cannot be successfully developed.

4.2.d Consequences

Structures that were previously insufficiently adapted to the here and now are completely overloaded by the extra burden of a systemic change coming from outside. The structural inability to interpret new situations and implement adequate action patterns quickly leads to an overload of statically relevant components of personality architecture - the vulnerability increases and as a result the extent of damage in the inter- and intra-personal space.

As a therapeutic approach, the concept of Personality After-ripening comes into consideration.

Until now was the assumption that personality development is substantially finished with the end of puberty - the individual then with its basic assumptions, the worldview and his experience largely unchangeable. This assumption was based on a biologistic approach, namely that the neuroplasticity decreases after puberty and new impressions and experiences that can hardly change "hardware".

Recent results have shown, however, that the brain after puberty quite well retains a corresponding neuro-plasticity. This is the basis for the concept of after-ripening. By fostering introspection ability and targeted levels of external effect issues such as self-awareness, empathy, self-image and social interaction skills are specifically formed. When the setting takes into account the operational requirements of an Asperger's patient, then he can benefit well (see chapter V "Psychotherapeutic Practice") - perhaps even better, because the whole thing needs an appropriate intellectual level.

4.3 Narcissistic Personality Structure

Like a Dissociated, also a Narcissistic Personality structure must be originally regarded and respected as adaptive.

Generally seen, narcissism (from the analytical point of view) is a response to the already experienced and therefore again feared for the future fright of losing a loved reference object. A strong personality architecture (i.e. typically already differentiated and adult) can allow this fear, possibly even show it adequately outward and handle it.

A weaker personality, for example, a child in his early years, feels this loss as an existential threat, which it has nothing to counter to. In order therefore to be able to (= neurotic) cope with that indirectly, it starts to devalue the reference object a priori and revalue himself to keep the damage to himself to a minimum in case of loss of relationship.

This procedure can be found in AS-people as a kind of coping strategy to regulate the relationship management for them perceived anyway as difficult to control, often highly hurtful.

Under the perspective of the SOC, there is a reversal of the proper order of comprehensibility, manageability and meaningfulness. The own importance is set as a postulate in the first place. From this then areas will be deduced and one focuses on those that are understandable and manageable at least in manageable limits.
A pseudo-comprehensibility and -manageability respectively a rigid SOC develops.

„Rigid SOC / strong SOC: The person with a rigid SOC holds to Koestler's canon respectively Gatlin's stored information. The person with a strong SOC looks for a balance between rules and strategies, between cached and potential information. It trusts that something meaningful can be done with the new information. It hardly feels a danger in regarding the world as a challenge and being open to feedback." [Antonovsky 1997]

In contrast to the behavior in a strong SOC people with a NPS respectively a Pseudo SOC are characterized by:

1. It is not man with NPS suffering, but his environment. Therefore, it comes to a diagnosis not until the narcissism building collapses.
2. They build their own narcissism-world in which they are the good guys, even the best. (significance)
3. In order to preserve this world, all conflicting events, expressions etc. will be ignored. This leads to a very limited perception of reality with a pronounced intolerance of other opinions and dissenters. (manageability)
4. Confrontations frequently occur by attacks at the relationship level - not at the factual level.
5. Alternatives or perspectives are not developed because they threaten the own, the pseudo-SOC-creative, vision of the world.
   Especially the normally existing skills of autistic people like solution orientation and interest may disappear almost completely. (comprehensibility)
6. People with NPS often criticize in order to protect their own vision of the world (at the relationship level), but are over-sensitive when being criticized themselves.
7. Self-criticism and rational self-assessment are largely lacking.

Particularly in the self-advocacy scene many autistic with severe narcissistic personality structure can be found. These then indeed demand integration and inclusion as normal people, but this please also without any outside criticism. Their conduct and statements, whether in blogs or forums, in books or magazines, in principle, are defined as perfect and not to be criticized. The self-contradictory demand for a "normal special role" is asserted.

So thanks to the involvement in the self-advocacy scene a pseudo-significance is achieved, however, in most cases, in fact, only in a very limited perception-bubble. A real external effect, there is little, because an open confrontation with the environment does not take place. At the same time frequently occurs a mutual acknowledgment within a small group of autism activists. Because autistic with NPS are strongly over-represented in the public and therefore in the public perception in relation to the entire autistic population, there may be a shift in perception of autism.

From an initially adaptive personality structure in the course of life almost inevitably develops a narcissism trap that leads to a reduction of the life and experience, namely, to the small circle of possible comprehensibility and manageability. As a result of this (self-)criticism is also excluded and so a salutogenic personal development as a whole is at least made difficult - if not prevented. Also, a NPS can mask an underlying autism so strongly, that this will be easily overlooked in the psychotherapeutic practice.

V. PSYCHOTHERAPEUTIC PRACTICE

For therapeutic practice at least three areas arise, to be discussed here in detail. Firstly, the creation of a barrier-free access, moreover the two questions of how autistic people can be detected without diagnosis and which therapeutic aims and methods are possible and meaningful in autism with or without diagnosis.

Recognizing autistic people without diagnosis in practice is of particular importance:

„At the same time in such studies a high probability was proven to develop secondary psychological disorders in the context of an autistic basic problem.
Given these aspects is understandable that certainly already far more people as perhaps previously believed with high-functioning autism are in psychotherapy.
[highlighting by the authors] And this often without themselves or the attending medical specialist or doctor knowing the autistic basic problem. This results in considerable problems arising - for all involved, but also for the supply system as a whole." [Wilczek 2015]

Example Consultation:
In a couple therapy, the autistic person is not recognized as such. Therefore, the possibilities of understanding as well as of positive changes remain in the dark. The couple therapy fails.

Example Clinic:
See Appendix, Case Report 1

The new development-dynamic perspective with diathesis-stress model should thereby facilitate the identification of autistic people. In any case, extensive knowledge about autism is of central importance for therapeutically active people.
In addition to undiagnosed autistic people which already (unrecognized) are in therapeutic treatment, there are many who have problems due to sensory hypersensitivity and / or anxiety disorders, to visit a practice. Some aspects in practice organization may represent hurdles for autistic people and obstruct the way to therapeutic support. Important is also to provide a preferably barrier-free access.

1 Accessibility

Because of the problematic psychotherapeutic provision in Germany, with long waiting lists, the following points appear naive and illusory. If demand exceeds the psychotherapeutic offers by far, the willingness to allow

accessibility for autistic people will be low. Because of
the size of the group (about 400,000 people in Germany)
and the growing psychological problems of autistic
people it nevertheless would be important. Especially
with regard to the previously mentioned study on the
increased mortality risk of autistic people - particularly
by suicide.

1.1   Appointment by Email

Many autistic have problems with telephoning. A contact
and appointment via email here is a great as well as easy
to be realized step towards accessibility.

1.2   Consideration of Hypersensitivity

A therapeutic interaction needs a preferably relaxing and
stress-free environment. However, the hypersensitivity is
the cause of stress and distraction in people with autism.
So paying attention to the sensory peculiarities of autistic
is important, because even something like a loud ticking
clock might make it difficult for the autistic clients to
concentrate. Considerations must include the full
spectrum of sensory perception.

1.2.a Visual

Disturbing is too bright lighting, as well as flickering light e.g. of defective neon lights. The clearer the environment, the less distracting and disturbing visual elements in the treatment room are available, the better.

1.2.b Auditory

All sounds are particularly strongly perceived by autistic and disturbing noises, like a ticking clock will not automatically be filtered out from perception. You have to keep an eye on a correspondingly quiet environment. A practice under the flight path of the airport, for example, is not a suitable place for the treatment of autistic.

1.2.c Olfactory

As stated, the odor perception of autistic is very sensitive. Strong odors are perceived as unpleasant. The practice, as well as the therapist himself should therefore be as odorless as possible.

1.3 Home Visits

Due to the insufficient supply it is a utopia, but home visits for many autistic would be the appropriate means. In case of heavy anxiety disorders and / or a total withdrawal from live an autistic will not be able to go to a practice.

As a consequence, therapeutic intervention will only begin when a (forced) admission due e.g. to a suicide attempt takes place. And that definitely is too late!

In addition, the domestic environment is familiar and therefore stress-free. Therapeutic efforts are therefore not hindered by anxiety and stress, or lack of energy, because this has been consumed for the way to practice. In future a close cooperation between administrative agencies, social workers and psychotherapists to ensure the best possible care would be desirable.

2 Anamnesis and Diagnosis

Both the detection of previously undiagnosed autistic and the knowledge about the active mechanisms to the development of mental disorders and structures which we have previously shown are important for the success of therapeutic intervention:

„If an autistic basic problem and the resulting differences is not recognized, so if the psychotherapist - and with him perhaps even the client - as described above assumes that the usual parameters and methods apply equally to him and would take effect like with any other, neuro-typical people, the symptoms mostly will not improve. In many cases, the secondary disturbances even

worsen as the central experience of "otherness" and the inability to be able to make comprehensible to others, again is confirmed - yes they are even aggravated by the impression, even in psychotherapy situation to be "somehow different" and "wrong" just to be "not good enough" respectively not understood." [Wilczek 2015]

If a diagnosis of autism is made, it requires the observance of some aspects.

2.1 With Asperger Diagnosis

As illustrated in people with autism somatic problems like eczema, gastrointestinal problems, back pain and headaches / migraines, dental problems ... go hand in hand with anxiety, stress and mental health problems. These somatic problems can thus serve as an indicator of the level of anxiety and stress, and also on behalf of the effectiveness of therapeutic intervention.

However, an investigation by medical specialists for causes is always required! Due to barriers, which in typical medical practices are even more distinctive, autistic usually tend to avoid medical consultations with corresponding negative consequences for health. Close cooperation between psychotherapists and specialists is therefore urgently needed. For information by specialists about the specifics of the treatment of autistic people and creating a barrier-free access, please refer to Schmidt, Ganz (2016) „*Klartext kompakt. Das Asperger Syndrom – für Ärzte*" as well as to

    www.barrierefrei.online (*German Website*)

Here you can find, inter alia, also current treatment guidelines for medical specialists as well as psychotherapists.

The treatment guideline may also serve to identify autistic people without actual diagnosis as such and configure the psychotherapeutic intervention accordingly.

2.2 Without Asperger Diagnosis

Recognizing an autism spectrum condition at a client is, as stated, of central importance. Here, inter alia, the inference of the existence of said somatic problems and the causes anxiety and stress can serve as an indicator of autism.

If in the anamnesis also problems with the unconscious group communication become apparent, a clarification of the Autism suspicion is required in any case.

2.3 SOC Questionnaire

To determine the SOC of the clients the questionnaire of Antonovsky with 29 items is useful.

For this, along with a scoring sheet please see:

www.barrierefrei.online (*German Website*)

In an online survey study conducted by us (n = 25) using the SOC questionnaire, the average SOC was at Asperger and highly functional autistic at only 103 points.

The German standardization of SOC-scale from the year 2000, however, gave an average value of 145 points (see Bengel et al. 2001). The SOC value of autistic individuals is therefore, as predicted, well below the average population value!

Measured by us lowest value was 57 points.

The highest SOC value was 130 points and thus still well below the normalized average.

„The sense of coherence shows a high negative correlation to dimensions of mental health such as anxiety and depression; i.e. people who have a high SOC are less anxious and depressed than people with a low SOC value."

[Bengel et al. 2001]

The inclusion of the SOC questionnaire as an additional diagnostic tool for AS-people therefore seems helpful.

3   Psychotherapy Procedures

The socio-psychological perspective and thus the perception of (the absence) of the unconscious group communication have far-reaching implications for psychotherapeutic intervention. Observing that there is no unconscious communication between client and therapist by mirroring and synchronization means that the therapeutic settings must be clearly different than in the case of NT people.

This also means that even psychotherapists first of all expect an unconscious relationship communication and can misinterpret the absence as rudeness or rejection. The limited communication and feedback from the AS-client can be misconstrued as a lack of cooperation. Communication with the client should be as concise and clear as possible in every case. You can, for example, orientate yourself on the title of this book - plaintext compact.

The verbal feedback to the client should be significantly more pronounced. Because the autistic client does not notice unconscious feedback and cannot decrypt this due to lack of autopilot.

An explicit and comprehensive feedback is therefore necessary.

Due to lack of participation in social interaction and communication the "common ground" necessary to communicate also often is not enough developed. This can lead to misunderstandings, as allusions are not understood and remarks of the therapist are taken literally. This requires a special sensitivity of the therapist.

Furthermore information and targeted procedures and processes are to be structured and visualized as well as possible, for example, by diagrams. AS people often have a visual thinking and can therefore better absorb respective information.

Also becomes clear that more likely cognitive therapies are suitable for autistic.
And that also the question of "significance", i.e. the question of "why at all?" should be answered, for example, by existential psychotherapy.

By the socio-psychological perspective and the resulting new perspective of interpersonal genesis of mental structures and disturbances in autism becomes clear that a classical therapy e.g. is of anxiety disorders, depression, narcissistic personality structure etc. is necessary but not sufficient. In order to be successful and, above all, be durable, the classical therapeutic approaches require supplementing with socio-psychological elements. This will be presented in the following again using the concept of salutogenesis by Antonovsky.

4 Goals of Therapy

Psychotherapy as a way to (mental) health goes well with Antonovsky's salutogenesis. In that exactly is shown as necessary for the development of health, what autistic just too often are lacking:
1. The ability to understand the relationships of life. The sense of comprehensibility.
2. The belief that one can make one's life. The sense of manageability.
3. The belief that life has meaning. The feeling of meaningfulness.

Also we have already shown the need for load balancing within the meaning of salutogenesis.

4.1 Load Balance – Reduction of Fear and Stress

In order to achieve a load balance, both the reduction of anxiety and stress and the buildup of resources for increasing the threshold are necessary.

Without default mode and instead having increased sensory sensitivity AS people are in a permanently increased state of excitement. The accompanying teaching of relaxation techniques is thus one of the important components of a successful therapy.

More specifically the means of reducing anxiety and stress, as well as development of resources are displayed in Schmidt (2015/2) „*Support for Autistic?*".

For children and adolescents also and especially the interaction with parents is to be taken into account. Parental involvement is therefore an urgent need! The influence of parents and their behavior to the development of autistic children can hardly be overestimated. So, for example, shows a study that learning mindfulness meditation by the parents (!) led to a dramatic improvement in the behavior of autistic children [Singh et al. (2014)].

4.2   Buildup of „Sense of Coherence"

Following the concept of salutogenesis, according to which the "sense of coherence" SOC in the form of the feeling of comprehensibility, manageability and meaningfulness is necessary for the development of health, the establishment of a SOC as a target stands in the foreground. But is a (low) SOC ever changeable and, if so, then how? Antonovsky is not optimistic on this issue and says:

„*The possibility of intentional modification: ... that without very significant, almost radical changes in the institutional, social and cultural settings that shape the life experiences of people it is utopian to expect that a meeting or even a series of encounters between the client and the clinician significantly alter the SOC. The own worldview that has formed over decades, is a too deeply rooted phenomenon, as it could be changed in such encounters."* [Antonovsky 1997]

However Antonovsky neither had in mind a psychotherapeutic intervention nor the peculiarities of perception and communication of autistic people. Therefore, we do not want to share Antonovsky's negative view, even if certainly often *"radical changes in ...the social ... ... settings"* will be necessary. So how can the SOC be strengthened and increased?

By the buildup of
1. Comprehensibility
2. Manageability
3. Significance

4.2.a   Comprehensibility

So far autistic had two problems with the sense of comprehensibility. On the one hand, that the other people are so different. This autistic hitherto often called and still call "Wrong Planet" syndrome. So the feeling of living on

the wrong planet, the rules and structures of which are not comprehensible.
On the other hand also, that there up to now has been no explanation, why this is so, what the difference is at all. There was a lack of an explanation on the meta-level.

Statement of an Autistic:
I will never understand my autism.

Due to the new socio-psychological perspective comprehensibility at least on the meta-level now is possible! The note of both the difference in sensory perception and the unconscious group communication respectively its absence will open access to the development of the sense of comprehensibility. Reading the books „*Understanding Autism*" (Schmidt 2015/1) and „*Support for Autistic?*" (Schmidt 2015/2) in practice has proven to have a positive impact on the development of comprehensibility with adults.
Only on the basis of comprehensibility, as described, a development of the feeling of manageability is reasonably possible.
The next questions to be answered, therefore, are how problems with the sense of manageability occur and can be prevented or stopped. So how to build up a sense of manageability.

4.2.b Manageability

How dramatically, at least in individual cases the attainment of comprehensibility can work directly onto the manageability, shall be described briefly:

Example Consultation:
A in spite of efforts hitherto not respectively misdiagnosed autistic understood after reading the social-psychological explanation approach both the reasons for her problems in the interaction and communication, as well as the difference between autism and her anxiety disorders and depressions. The autistic then terminates her THC consumption, deliberately dismounts her anxiety disorders and is looking for social contacts. The emotional instability previously misdiagnosed as borderline is reduced and a dramatic improvement in the overall situation taking place within weeks, for example, inter alia, by now consistent (so far avoided) visit of doctors e.g. for checkups.

Unfortunately there is not always such rapid and significant improvement due to a new understanding of one's own situation. In the example we are on the one hand at Stage 2, i.e. problems caused by anxiety and stress, but without trauma(ta) exceeding the stress threshold border(s). Also it can be assumed that underlying a high SOC existed, which has been updated.

Where a basic high SOC does not exist, it is important to take into consideration and to promote three areas for improvement. This is the only way to secure a long-term success of therapeutic intervention.

1.) Building Social (!) Contacts in Task Mode

Social contacts are essential components for the construction of comprehensibility, as the basis of self-esteem and also as a resource to support the sense of manageability. However, most contact options are based on the default mode including unconscious group communication, gossip. Attempts to contact will fail in such structures already due to the ingroup / outgroup distinction and autistic as "no-group" (see Schmidt 2015/1).

Possible, however, are social contacts into groups, which are essentially clearly structured and mainly act in task mode.

Mention may be made here, for example, of Repair Cafes, organizations such as THW (German technical social aid), fire fighters …

2.) Change of Environment Instead of Withdrawal

Detours always increase the local knowledge, and so is the change of a sensory not tolerable environment, for example, in a big city, be preferred to the whereabouts.

A correspondingly less exiting (living-) environment can contribute much to the positive development.
And especially when the social environment permanently shows negative reactions e.g. in the form of bullying or exclusion, a change of this environment is strongly advised.

„Of particular importance are our social networks which in research are proven to have resource status. We make over the years - apart from primary relationships with parents, siblings, relatives, and later with work colleagues - our self-selected networks by developmentally learning to decide, with whom we want to spend our lives and how long, who we want to have around us. But freedom of decision given to us will, however, reach its limits where we at times have to submit to massive physical and social constraints to ever have access to the resources. Undoubtedly people who can live social interaction on the basis of a mutual give and take have an advantage: They participate in social support for perceived challenges of their lives as are to cope with in everyday incidences, so even in crises, by recourse to particular idle resources. Suffering can be shared by communication, as analogously stated in a famous saying, therefore the sympathy of caregivers with which we can exchange about our loss experience,

develops its strength as one of the most important coping resources on which we can fall back." [Lorenz 2005]

As hard as the change respectively acquiring of a new social environment may be, as necessary it is at the same time.
Thus understood we agree with Antonovsky when he says, *„...that without very significant, almost radical changes in the institutional, social and cultural settings that shape the life experiences of people it is utopian to expect that a meeting or even a series of meetings between the client and the clinician can significantly alter the SOC."* [Antonovsky 1997]

3.) Work
The third central area for developing a sense of manageability is work.
„The third variable to be considered is the type of social relations within the working group. To the extent in which there are common values, a sense of group identification and unambiguous normative expectations, the atmosphere will be characterized by consistency. In such a setting one will always receive adequate feedback. One sends signals and knows that they are understood, as well as one understands the signals that are sent. Symbols are shared; there is a common language. To the

outsider, things may seem chaotic for the insider they are not. Group rituals amplify the experience of the consistency." [Antonovsky 1997]

However, many studies show that only about 1/3 of diagnosed autistic find an adequate work. The majority is either unemployed or despite normal to high intelligence is found in sheltered workshops or precarious employment. Since autistic additionally always are in task mode, are problem solvers and are interested, work has a very special status.

Example Clinic:
See Appendix, Case Report 2

Reality however in a DM-oriented affluent society is somewhat different. In many fields of work today so-called "soft skills" in the sense of (unconscious) group behavior are important, that is, that in working groups the unconscious level predominates.
„In any group of individuals, which comes together with a certain purpose, there is a conscious, task-oriented group and an underlying, unconscious group; the functioning of this underlying group may be in conflict with the requirements of the task. This is not to say that working groups will never work. We are from a variety of

reasons - work, politics, interests and free time - members in groups and we mostly manage to accomplish their tasks. However, the performance may be affected by fears, which we perhaps are not aware of, and by processes that develop in the group to reduce anxieties."
[Wetherell 1996]

In particular, activities which often demand and encourage pronounced problem-solving ability and creativity from AS-people, would be important for autistic to build a sense of manageability.

„ ... Kohn und Schooler (1983) on substantial complexity. They showed for various dimensions of personality, also including the experience of distress, which long-term effects arise depending on the extent to which the jobs require substantive complexity, in order to exercise them appropriately. Although their discussion neglects the risk of too much complexity there is little doubt that for too many people - and this is first and foremost for minorities, women and people with disabilities - the absence of substantive complexity of work, which does not consider their potentials is leading to increasing paralysis of their experience of manageability."
[Antonovsky 1997]

Therefore the client's taking up an adequate employment (if not existent) is necessary not only for obtaining financial independence but also for the development of the feeling of manageability. To facilitate this and to pave the way at employers see also „*Klartext kompakt. Das Asperger Syndrom für Arbeitgeber*" [Schmidt (2016/1)]. A corresponding cooperation with advisory centers, social and psychological services and integration advisors here would be helpful and desirable.

4.2.c   Significance

The stigma of "failure" and the deficit-oriented and pathologizing perspective so far has been detrimental to the development of the feeling of meaningfulness in autism. So important are especially the abandonment of deficit orientation and instead acceptance and compliance with existing strengths! And that both in the social as well as in the scientific field!
And also experienced marginalization and exclusion of "socially accepted decision-making processes" hitherto prevents the feeling of meaningfulness.
„Participating in socially accepted decision-making processes also provides us with the opportunity to identify with the events. It causes that we can experience our actions as significant. To the extent in which we and our actions are seen by others and identified with it, the

feeling of importance will experience consolidation. The goal is always to realize your own intentions, to influence and to convey decisions." [Lorenz 2005]

Unfortunately autistic altogether were and are, rather than being involved in decision-making processes, paternalistically patronized. And this even and especially by aid structures. Hitherto also there, participation, which is usual, is ignored. But even after a recommendation of the Bavarian Districts assembly from 2015 to implement a participation structure in government funded autism institutions, these still do not exist.
But a participation in decision making must repeatedly be demanded and first of all implemented.

As a further point to build significance the change away from a deficit and towards a strength orientation is to be mentioned. This also applies to the understanding of autism and autistic clients by the therapist.
Already in 1999, Carol Gray and Tony Attwood have published the "Criteria for the discovery of Aspie" (The text is freely available in the internet at multiple locations).
The approach was to define and to rediscover Asperger's Syndrome not by deficits, but by positive features.

As qualitative benefits Gray & Attwood mentioned, among other things:

In the field of <u>social interaction</u>:
- Peer relationships characterized by absolute loyalty and impeccable reliability.
- Free of prejudice on grounds of sex, age or culture; ability to accept others as they are.
- Expresses his own thoughts irrespective of social context or sticks to personal convictions.

In the field of <u>cognitive abilities</u>:
- Original, often unique way of solving problems.
- Exceptional memory and / or remembrance of details that are often forgotten or ignored by others, such as names, dates, schedules, routines.
- Enthusiastic perseverance in collecting and collating information about a topic of interest.
- Persistence of thinking.

And <u>additionally</u>:
- Socially "unsung hero" with trusting optimism: frequent victim of social weaknesses of others and still clinging to the belief that real friendships are possible.

- A higher probability than in the general population, to attend university after high school.
- Often caring towards others outside the scope of typical development.

Unfortunately, however, this view has been adopted neither by the research nor by society.
They instead remain at a purely deficit perspective. But one is autistic a lifetime and the sense of importance can only be generated if the strengths of autistic are seen and (can be) developed in an unfavorable socio-cultural environment.

„The motivational component of significance appears to be most important. Without it a high degree of comprehensibility and manageability is likely to be of short duration. The person, who is committed and cares, has the possibility to gain understanding and resources. Comprehensibility seems to be in order of importance in the next place, because a high degree of manageability depends on the understanding. That does not mean that manageability is unimportant. If you do not believe that resources are available, the significance decreases, and coping efforts become weaker. Successful coping therefore depends on the SOC as a whole."
[Antonovsky 1997]

So the psychological problems of autistic arise from the interaction with a more or less favorable environment. And psychotherapy takes place in a socio-cultural environment, which can certainly massively impede the positive development and successful therapeutic intervention - and up to date because of pathologizing and deficit orientation even does so. Here a quick and profound change by the commitment of all stakeholders is necessary. But even with autistic clients there are special antagonisms that may be in the way of an initiation of therapy respectively its successful implementation. These are primarily special forms of anxiety avoidance behavior in people with autism.

5 Antagonism: „Anxiety Avoiding Behavior"

In social-psychology has long been known that (unconscious) group behavior is also and above all to avoid anxiety. Without the ability to participate in unconscious group behavior, autistic thus lack this possibility of avoiding anxiety. What NT people accomplish as a group, autistic people must each make for themselves. All are whistling in the dark forest, but NT people in the choir, autistic however alone. This frequently leads in people with autism to three for therapeutic intervention possibly problematic behaviors.

5.1 Avoidance of Change

„*Avoidance of change: Change is an excursion into the unknown. It means a commitment to future events that are not entirely predictable, as well as their consequences, and inevitably calls forth doubts and fears. Any significant change in a social system brings with it changes in the existing social relations and in the social structure, which in turn leads to the fact that the effectiveness of the social system as a protection system changes ... To avoid these fears, the service tried to avoid changes as far as possible, and to cling to the familiar, even if the familiar obviously no longer was appropriate or relevant.*" [Menzies Lyth (1960)]

Autistic often exhibit a particularly pronounced form of avoiding change. And this particularly at high anxiety and stress levels. A reduction of anxiety and stress as well as the formation of the feelings of comprehensibility and manageability have to come first.

5.2 Intolerance of Uncertainty

Also in people with autism often a massive intolerance to uncertainty is found. The predictive planning of all activities then has top priority.
The client should therefore be informed as

comprehensive and as early as possible about further proceedings.

5.3 Insistence on Sameness

The third point to mention is the insistence on uniformity (sameness). Any change of processes, practices, the environment, etc. creates fear and is avoided. Here again the reduction of anxiety and stress and the development of feelings of comprehensibility and manageability must come first. This -and that should be clear to the therapist- can be a long burdensome way for the patience of the therapist. Quite easily with people with autism "cannot" is confused with "does not want".

VI. EPILOGUE

Goal of the series "plaintext compact" is not a comprehensive description of all aspects of Asperger syndrome, but the mediation of the new social-psychological, and developmental dynamic perspective. So this book essentially should open new doors, open perspectives and show directions.

However, the concrete ways of therapeutic interaction are manifold. Using the examples of "learned helplessness" of Seligman and "salutogenesis" by Antonovsky possible applications of the new perspectives were highlighted. In summary is to reemphasize that autistic people have a high vulnerability to the development of mental disorders, the HRQL often being low and the risk of suicide high. So far autistic are however often not, too late or incorrectly diagnosed. An increased sensitivity regarding a possible autism spectrum structure with clients is therefore just as urgent as the creation of a barrier-free access. To influence also the environment and e.g. to stop bullying, cooperation with counseling centers, social services etc. in case of need is to be sought.

VII. APPENDIX

Case Report 1

Anamnesis:

The patient (20 years) on a Sunday morning is admitted to the emergency room of a psychiatric acute care clinic after a suicide attempt attended by his parents. According to the parents (the patient at this time refused to communicate with the medical staff) the patient's girlfriend had told him the night before via Skype that she ends the relationship. This in the light of the fact, that for of kinship reasons she wanted to return to the United States and he did not want to accompany her. The girlfriend had been the only attachment figure outside the family for years.

After the news he had retired to his room - the next morning the mother had noticed cuts on his wrists, so she and her partner could -despite significant resistance- ultimately move the patient to hospitalization.

No stationary pretreatments, for years psycho-pharmacological treatment with antidepressants (duloxetine), formerly temporarily treated with methylphenidate by the child and adolescent psychiatrist due to an ADHD diagnosis.

Admittance Situation:
In the initial contact situation there is a physically healthy age-appropriate man. Clothing more functional, avoiding eye contact, standing at the wall in the receiving room. Tensely psycho-motorized. On the question of the doctor on duty, whether the conversation should be continued without the parents present, this is clearly affirmed.

After collecting psychopathological findings which besides an affective reduction and a significantly reduced resilience showed no trendsetting pathologic, especially no acute suicidality.

Subsequent Course:
After an acute self- and other hazard may be ruled out, the patient is transferred to an open psychotherapy station.
For clarification on suspicion of Asperger's syndrome, the reference psychologists used the Adult Asperger Assessment by (Baron-Cohen et al., German version AAA D, translated and supplemented by Christine M. Freitag and Kathrin Leistenschneider). Inquired were the areas of social interaction, special interests, communication and imagination.

Appendix

The AAA-D was carried out both as a structured interview, as well as evaluated with recourse to the responses of the patient to the questionnaires for the Autism Spectrum Quotient (AQ;. Baron-Cohen et al, 2001) and Empathy Quotient (EQ; Baron- Cohen et al., 2004). The questionnaire information referred to significant impairments in all investigated areas except the imagination. The interview data and the behavioral observation allowed a differentiated view of the symptomatology:

The social interaction appeared normal at first glance. The nonverbal behavior was normal. In contact with other patients, the patient was very articulate, appeared extroverted, stepped up to others and quickly found connection. In everyday life, there are friendships with peers. The patient himself described, he enjoyed spending time in company, but this was also tiring, he accordingly had a clear need for rest and relaxation. He was basically nice to people, but he felt an inner distance, was hardly emotionally capable of oscillating, experiencing his emotional behavior more like a simulation of appropriate emotion. Friends seemed interchangeable in most cases. The patient was for many people a figure of trust and got feedback to react very supportive and appropriate.
He himself regards this capability as learned. He reserved

his own problems other hand, mostly for himself, in the expectation of being not understood anyway. In the stationary frame was observed that he often played the role of a co-therapist, appeared outwardly very confident and hardly dissembled uncertainties. With regard to the interpretation of social situations he often was uncertain, expecting rejection and therefore apparently questioning friendly behavior of his opponent. Only through physical contact he could directly experience affection.

In discussions he was accused of representing his own position too one-sided or vehemently. He finds it difficult in such situations, to take a different view than his own. Also he often gets a feedback on a pedantic narrative style. About his interests he spoke to some extent excessively detailed. Personal conversation he would mostly exclude, he had no interesting inner life, worth telling.

Moreover was reported back to him that he was often undiplomatic. The patient utters his opinion, even if he could criticize or hurt others. This he accepted mostly consciously.
But he was sometimes uncertain whether a joke was still acceptable, or could seem offensive or inappropriate.

The patient is very interested in tactical PC games and fantasy culture (Yu-Gi-Oh cards (a complex TCG), Cosplay, novels example of S. King). He was involved in a circle of friends who shares these interests.

Own medical history on the development only exist in an insufficient extent. The patient hardly remembers events before age 12. In kindergarten, the patient was well integrated. In the second and third year of primary school, he had then lost many friends by deliberately harming behavior. Even towards his parents he had been very hurtful. A foreign history is recommended, however, was initially postponed due to priority therapy areas of focus.

The patient fully participated in the offered psychotherapy program with psychoanalytically oriented individual and group therapy, among others on depression management, employment and creative therapy, music therapy, exercise, sports and fitness therapy, dance therapy, psychosomatic ward and attendant care in the nursing team, participating in the patient community with acceptance of various tasks, learning a relaxation method (autogenous training) and disorder-specific behavioral interventions.

The initial depressed mood soon changed into a depressed feeling of numbness. A pattern of habitual emotion avoidance and self-invalidation became clear that was classified biographically later in therapy. In therapy, the patient dealt with his emotional and social experience and behavior and made corrective relationship experiences (to be taken seriously, to be understood, to be liked, to give and take). As part of an extremely changeable course with in the meantime significant deterioration of the condition his mood and drive finally improved, the capacity for joy returned. The patient now could consider concrete targets and thus developed a life perspective.

Following the stay a temporary day hospital treatment and beyond the implementation an ambulant psychotherapy is recommended.

Case Report 2

Situation First Contact:
Emergency allocation per provisional accommodation decision because of endangerment after prior notification by a family doctor colleague. Patient is said to have attacked a roommate with a butter knife in the facility where he is housed since a year.

Patient arrives about 15 minutes later, accompanied by two paramedics. He avoids eye contact in the welcome situation. But in the following conversation in a receiving space well examinable, no evidence of self-harm or hazard. In the communication part telegram-like expression; however, an intercurrently reoccurring tendency to monologues on various topics, sometimes barely interruptible (on attempts to interrupt him the patient casually raises "not now!") is to be noticed. When asked about the background of the incident in the home, he indicates that the roommate disturbed him since his arrival in the facility during drying, which he procures every day since his admission 13 months ago. To verbal delineation he did not react, therefore this measure would have been necessary for him to have peace again.

Anamnesis/ External medical history:
21 year old patient. For one year now housed at a facility in the vicinity. Attendance of the special school to the age of 17, afterwards working in a sheltered workshop. Parents divorced, no contact with the father, regular contact with the mother and the younger sister. Reception reason in the socio-therapeutic residential group of the facility: increasing health restriction of the mother, where the patient had lived until then.

The patient as described by the mother has always been very reclusive, neither in kindergarten nor in school contacts with peers. Could already read before enrollment; but in school significant deficits, so from 3rd year following the advice of the primary school teacher at a special school. Recurring outbreaks of violence against peers in the school sector.
After the end of the school career Transfer into a sheltered workshop near the home of the mother, and later inclusion in an affiliated residential group.
At home, the patient had mostly stayed in his room, hobbies were reading and "tinkering geometric figures".

Psycho-dynamic Anamnesis:
In several exploratory meetings the patient talks about his biographical career. He had never particularly been interested in his peers, as they would have barely been interested in things that were important to him. In kindergarten he had preferably viewed picture books; after he had taught himself the alphabet, he had begun to decipher the individual words, thereby he had learned to read. He could write only much later, since the implementation of the letters on paper long had been difficult. The kindergarten teachers had tried to "force" him into contact to other children by taking away the books. During this time it often came to aggressive

behavior towards other children if they did not want to leave him in peace. Thereafter, the kindergarten teachers had always accused him to be responsible.

Later, the situation had continued in school; team sports as ball games etc. were experienced particularly unpleasant.

He felt most comfortable when he could pursue his self-chosen occupations, having his rest and the day being planned.

In the facility that mostly went well, however, a new roommate some time ago had come into his residential group, who by his agitated behavior had caused the patient a strong stress increase. As on the morning of the day of reception he had repeatedly disturbed him when drying cutlery and had become loud, he did not take it anymore and tried to expel him with a butter knife, hoping to keep him permanently at a distance.

A supervisor had noticed this, so he had eventually entered the psychiatry.

During exploration some delicate objects from wooden sticks catch the eye, which the patient has produced in the ergo-therapy. On the casual question of the speaker, of what these depicted, the patient begins a nearly fifteen-minute statement in the field of theoretical physics, which was one of his hobbies. With regard to contents (to the extent the speaker can follow) stringently. In further

conversation there is another focus of interest in theoretical pharmacology, especially in the field of receptor / ligand - interaction.
These centers of interest are the mental main areas in which the patient is staying. In this area, things are meaningful, sensible, comprehensible and somehow controllable. All this is as it were a counterpart to the unpleasant chaotic, loud, aggressive and barren of inspiration environment.

Progress:
In the stationary frame, the patient showed no abnormalities, participated in the guided creative therapies with great interest, however, showed virtually no interest in the patient community.
Because of the strong scientific and pharmacological interest a taster internship at a local near pharmaceutical company for phytotherapy has been arranged, the department head of research was personally known to the speaker. This turned out to be surprisingly positive, so that after completion of the guide lined diagnosis, the patient was discharged not only into the old relations, but has been included into a regular traineeship in the company.

By further inquiry of the speaker after one year it was found that this internship was converted into a permanent position.

VIII. GLOSSARY

ASC	autism spectrum condition ; contrast to „disorder"
AS-Human	Human from the autism spectrum
DM	Default-Mode
Entropy	Movement of natural systems towards a state of maximum disorder.
fuzzy	blurry
NPS	narcissistic personality structure
NT-Human	Neuro-typical human
Salutogenesis	„way to health" contrast to pathogenesis
SOC	sense of coherence
TM	Task-Mode

IX. BIBLIOGRAPHY

Antonovsky, Aaron; Franke, Alexa (1997):
Salutogenese. Zur Entmystifizierung der Gesundheit.
Tübingen: DGVT-Verl. (36).
ISBN: 978-3871591365

Attwood, T., & Gray, C. (1999).
The Discovery of 'Aspie'Criteria.
In: The Morning News, 11(3).

Bargh, John A. (2014): Social psychology and the unconscious. The automaticity of higher mental processes.

Bengel, Jürgen; Strittmatter, Regine; Willmann, Hildegard (2001):
Was erhält Menschen gesund? Antonovskys Modell der Salutogenese - Diskussionsstand und Stellenwert ; eine Expertise.
Köln: BZgA (Forschung und Praxis der Gesundheitsförderung, 6).
Online verfügbar unter http://www.bzga.de/infomaterialien/forschung-und-praxis-der-gesundheitsfoerderung/band-06-was-erhaelt-menschen-gesund-antonovskys-modell-der-salutogenese/.
ISBN: 3933191106

Dell'Osso, Liliana; Dalle Luche, Riccardo; Carmassi, Claudia (2015):
A New Perspective in Post-Traumatic Stress Disorder: Which Role for Unrecognized Autism Spectrum?
In: International Journal of Emergency Mental Health and Human Resilience Vol. 17, No.2, S. 436–438.

Downey, Geraldine; Feldmann, Scott I. (1996):
Implications of Rejection Sensitivity für Intimate Relationships. In: Journal of Personality and Social Psychology (6), S. 1327–1343.

Hirvikoski, Tatja, et al. (2015):
Premature mortality in autism spectrum disorder.
In: The British Journal of Psychiatry

Lorenz, Rüdiger (2005):
Salutogenese. Grundwissen für Psychologen, Mediziner, Gesundheits- und Pflegewissenschaftler.
2., durchges. Aufl. München, Basel: E. Reinhardt.
ISBN: 3497016977

Menzies Lyth, Isabel (1960): Social Systems as a Defense Against Anxiety. An Empirical Study of the Nursing Service of a General Hospital. In: Human Relations (13), S. 95–121.

Schmidt, Bernhard J. (2015 / 1):
Autistic and Society - An angry change of perspective: Volume 1: Understanding Autism
1. Aufl. Norderstedt: Books on Demand.
ISBN: 978-3738634662

Schmidt, Bernhard J. (2015 / 2):
Autistic and Society - An angry change of perspective.: Volume 2: Support for Autistic?
1. Aufl. Norderstedt: Books on Demand.
ISBN: 978-3738655384

Schmidt, Bernhard J. (2016/1):
Klartext kompakt.
Das Asperger Syndrom - für Arbeitgeber.
1. Aufl. Norderstedt: Books on Demand.
ISBN: 978-3739228082

Schmidt, Bernhard J. (2016/2):
Klartext kompakt.
Das Asperger Syndrom –
Zwischen Mobbing und Inklusion
1. Aufl. Norderstedt: Books on Demand.
ISBN: 978-3839147917

Schmidt, Bernhard J.; Ganz, Andreas (2016):
Klartext kompakt. Das Asperger Syndrom - für Ärzte
1. Aufl. Norderstedt: Books on Demand.
ISBN: 978-3739240893

Seligman, Martin E. P. (1975):
Helplessness. On depression, development, and death.
San Francisco, New York: W.H. Freeman; Trade
distributor, Scribner. ISBN: 0716707519

Singh, Nirbhay N. et al. (2014):
Mindfulness-Based Positive Behavior Support (MBPBS)
for Mothers of Adolescents with Autism Spectrum
Disorder: Effects on Adolescents' Behavior and Parental
Stress. In: Mindfulness 5 (6), S. 646–657.
DOI: 10.1007/s12671-014-0321-3.

Waterhouse, Lynn H. (Hg.) (2013): Rethinking autism.
Variation and complexity. 1st ed. London, Waltham, MA:
Academic Press.

Wetherell, Margaret (Hg.) (1996): Identities, groups and
social issues. London: SAGE.

Wilczek, Brit (2015):
Erwachsene mit hochfunktionalem Autismus in der psychotherapeutischen Praxis. Herausforderungen und Chancen. In: Psychotherapeutenjournal (2), S. 120–129.

Woods, Alisa G. (2013):
Bullying and Autism.
In: Autism 03 (03). DOI: 10.4172/2165-7890.1000e118.